Intermittent Fasting For Beginners

The complete guide to fat loss, better health, and a faster metabolism through intermittent fasting

Table of Contents

Introduction iv

Chapter 1 – What is Intermittent Fasting? 1

Chapter 2 – Intermittent Fasting: Benefits and Drawbacks 6

Chapter 3 – The 4 Most Popular Intermittent Fasting Protocols 10

Chapter 4 – Step-By-Step Guide to Intermittent Fasting 14

Chapter 5 – Three Common Mistakes Made by Beginners 18

Chapter 6 – Best Practices 21

Conclusion 26

Introduction

I want to thank you and congratulate you for downloading the book, *"Intermittent Fasting For Beginners"*.

This book contains helpful information about what intermittent fasting is, and how you can use it.

Intermittent fasting is rising to popularity quick, and for one simple reason – it works!

However, for intermittent fasting to work properly, you need to understand how to engage in it properly. Through reading this, you will soon discover a range of fasting methods that will help you achieve the health and fitness goals you are chasing!

This book will explain to you tips and techniques that will allow you to successfully change your diet and easily lose weight with intermittent fasting!

Thanks again for downloading this book, I hope you enjoy it!

Chapter 1 – What is Intermittent Fasting?

Obesity is one of the most persistent issues America has to face. The popularity of weight loss diet plans, pills, exercises, and fad diets only proves that there is a huge market for these weight loss regimens.

Fad diets can give you good results but they don't supply long term benefits. Luckily, there is an emerging "breakout diet plan" that is gaining more supporters. It is an unlikely regimen as it poses a challenge. It defies the belief the fasting as a form of dieting will actually make you gain more weight once the fasting period is done. However, intermittent fasting is different and it is fast gaining ground.

What is intermittent fasting?

Fasting simply means not eating. Intermittent fasting is alternately feeding and fasting. You set a specific schedule when you are to eat and not to eat. There are different "fasting periods" that are recommended, it can be a 16-hour period, 20-hour, 24-hour, or 36-hour period. There are people, who, because they want to get immediate weight loss results, resort to fasting; however, they fail to get the results they want because of the fact that they do not know the proper techniques to lose excess weight by fasting.

When you sleep, you fast, hence, the first meal when you wake up is called "breakfast" as it literally breaks your fasting period. If breakfast is the most important meal of the day, why does intermittent fasting tell you to skip it?

With intermittent fasting, you are not supposed to eat breakfast at all. For many years, you have been told that in order to get yourself going for the day's tasks, you need to eat breakfast, even more so if you want to lose weight.

Intermittent fasting is actually not a diet plan but simply a dieting pattern. You consciously skip certain meals. Meaning, you "fast and feast" on purpose, which means, you eat your calories at specific times of the day and opting not to eat food during the rest of the day. Since you are already fasting as you sleep, skipping breakfast allows you to extend your fasting time.

Two Ways to Take Advantage of Intermittent Fasting

- Regular eating for a specific time period. You prefer to eat only between the 12 noon and 8pm window, entirely skipping breakfast. There are people who choose to eat in a 4-hour window or a 6-hour window.

- Skipping 2 meals a day and having a 24-hour fasting period. You can eat on your normal eating schedule: you may be done with dinner at 8pm, and then fast until 8pm the next day.

You might think that if you skip a meal and eat less than what you normally eat, you can lose weight. This practice may or may not make you lose weight. You can skip a meal and consume the same amount of calories that you need, to stay healthy and fit, and still make you lose weight. But, it is important to take note that not all calories are the same, so the right timing is essential to intermittent fasting.

How Does Intermittent Fasting Work?

When you practice intermittent fasting to lose weight, your body reacts differently when you "feast" compared to the periods when you "fast". This is the reason why:

> When you eat a full meal, your body works for hours to process the foods, burning whatever you have consumed to be used as energy and nutrients. Your body will quickly burn the foods you just ate and convert to energy rather than store them as fat. When you eat carbohydrates and/or sugar, your body will immediately burn the sugar into energy before any other food.

> When you are on your "fasting period", your body doesn't have any available source of food to be converted to energy, so it will likely get from your fat storage, instead of actually utilizing the glucose present in your blood or the glycogen that your

muscles and liver produce. In effect, your body burns the fat you have stored in your body and you lose weight.

This principle is also true when you do your workout during the fasting stage. When there is an absence of readily available supply of glucose and glycogen (since you are in the fasting state), your body will be forced to adapt during the workout to get energy from the only available source, which is the stored fat in your cells.

This principle actually works! Why? Your body reacts to energy consumption (as you eat food) with the production of insulin. Your body becomes more sensitive to insulin, resulting to consuming food more efficiently, thus helping in weight loss and muscle development. Take note that your body is more sensitive to insulin after a fasting period.

Your body's glycogen level becomes depleted when you are sleeping (or during the fasting period), it will continue to decrease when you work out during the time that you are fasting, thus increasing your body's sensitivity to insulin. This can only mean one thing, the moment you eat after working out, the foods you consume will be efficiently stored: glycogen will go to your muscle storage, and fat is burned as energy to help in your body's recovery process, thus storing a very little amount of fat.

Think about it: if you are not intermittent fasting and your insulin level is maintained at its normal levels, the foods, especially carbohydrates, you consume will be stored as fat almost instantly and at increased levels.

Simply put, following intermittent fasting pattern teaches your body to utilize the foods you consume more efficiently.

Chapter 2 – Intermittent Fasting: Benefits and Drawbacks

Intermittent fasting, when done properly, can provide huge weight loss benefits. The concept of fasting for weight loss is not entirely new. It has been used by a lot of obese people who want to lose weight fast. However, if done incorrectly, you may lose weight quickly but then gain back all the weight you lost, and add more than what you lost, when you begin eating normally again. Consciously altering your eating patterns has its benefits and drawbacks. It must be done correctly to gain the benefits. You are not starving yourself, just focusing on eating at different times of the day, rather than eating constantly. Fasting also has different effects on different people, so what works for you might not work for other and vice versa.

The Benefits of Intermittent Fasting

1. **Detoxification**

   You may not be aware of it, but your body undergoes its own cleansing and detoxifying process all day. Your body is functioning the way it should be when it can easily identify and immediately replace worn out or damaged cells. This process is called autophagy. This is an ongoing and automatic process, but it can be jeopardized when you have a poor diet. However, a healthy diet can also slow the process down because when your body is digesting foods, the custodial duties of your cells are decreased.

Your body needs time to solely focus on cell repair. Autopaghy is increased during your fasting period, thus aiding in detoxification.

2. Helps regulate hormones

Fasting has a huge impact on the levels of your human growth hormones. An increase in the levels of your HGH will give you faster muscle repair, growth, and increased endurance, in addition to slowing down the aging process.

3. Promotes insulin sensitivity

As mentioned in the previous chapter, fasting allows for better use of foods by your body, and improves insulin sensitivity after a fasting period.

4. Leptin manipulation

Your leptin levels are decreased during the fasting period, but it gets a big boost when you begin to eat again.

5. It helps simplify your life

You don't have to prepare meals every 2 to 3 hours, thus saving you time and money. It also allows you to have more time for work, thus increasing your productivity, whether you need to do household chores or office tasks. Instead of preparing, cooking, and eating 6 times a day, you only need to prepare and cook meals as little as twice a day.

6. **It simply works!**

    Fasting gives your body the chance to lose weight since it puts your body in a state where it burns calories rather than storing them as fat deposits.

The Drawbacks of Intermittent Fasting

Proponents of intermittent fasting attest that it has very few negative side effects. One of the biggest concerns, though, is that you tend to have lower energy and less focus during your fasting period. There is also a huge concern about skipping breakfast and feeling lethargic the whole morning until you are able to eat for lunch.

These are common initial reactions of both your mind and your body. When you have been used to eating all the time, fasting can be a challenge during the first two weeks. However, when you get past the transition stage and your body has adapted well into the process, your body will be back to functioning normally.

Most of the time, your body's reaction to skipping breakfast can be traced back to your eating habits. It can also be because of mind conditioning. When you have been used to eating after every 3 hours, your body automatically becomes hungry every 3 hours and learns to expect to eat after short intervals. So, if your body has been used to eating breakfast, you will wake up feeling hungry and looking for food. You can safely say that everything is purely mental conditioning. Once your body becomes used to the intermittent fasting pattern, your body adapts and you only feel the hunger when it's time to eat.

When your body gets used to skipping breakfast, your morning grumpiness will also change because you have clearly adapted to the pattern.

Chapter 3 – The 4 Most Popular Intermittent Fasting Protocols

Feast/Fast

The feast/fast protocol can be considered as the most commonly used among the 8 intermittent fasting protocols. There is a "period of fasting" and a "period of feasting" or the cheat days. You can eat three full meals today and fast tomorrow (consuming only fluids), and so on.

Benefits: When you have limited food intake, leptin levels drop, slowing down fat loss. When you start eating after a fasting period, leptin levels increase, fast tracking fat loss. Leptin is the hormone produced by fat cells which is responsible in regulating the amount of fat that is to be stored in the body.

Drawbacks: You always have to do the "cheat days" or the days when you eat after a fasting period. There are some who don't like having the cheat days, thinking that it might jeopardize their weight-loss process. Cheat days actually help as much as the no-food days. The main discomfort is when you skip eating for extended periods, like 24 to 36 hours. If the discomfort bothers you, try to begin with a lesser period, like 16 to 18 hours and adjust when your body has adapted.

The 24-Hour Fasting Period (Eat-Stop-Eat)

As the name implies, you have to refrain from eating for 24 hours. If you had your last meal at 7pm on Sunday, you do not eat until Monday night, 7pm. You can do this 1 to 3 times a week.

Benefits: One their main benefits is that you can easily incorporate this intermittent fasting protocol to your own lifestyle. It's hard to miss this because you simply do not eat for 24 hours. This is easier to achieve than the 36-hour fast. It works because the absence of calorie-intake for extended periods aids in weight loss.

Drawbacks: Some people just cannot bring themselves to not eat for a 24-hour period. There are also those who have low blood sugar levels and to go on without food for longer periods won't work for them. If you are one of them, you have to consider taking shorter fasting periods.

The 20-Hour Fasting Period (Warrior Diet)

This method works by fasting for 20 hours and then eating during the 4-hour window. This is also called the "warrior diet" since it is patterned after the eating habits of the warriors of antiquity. Roman centurions of the old Roman Empire would eat one large meal for dinner and eat a small amount of foods for breakfast.

In most cases, a small breakfast and large dinner will work, but some people are skeptical because of the small amount of time between the 2 meals. There are even dieters who skip the breakfast meal and just stick with the large dinner meal in the hopes of maximizing the benefits of fasting.

Benefits: You can get the same benefits as doing the 24-hour fast method. This generally results in a lower calorie intake. You can eat anything for the large dinner, as long as you have the right amount of nutrients. You can even indulge in dessert and junk foods if you please, but not too much. In addition, having one large meal a day simplifies your life.

Drawbacks: The main issue is similar to the 24-hour fast since you will deprive yourself of food for longer periods. You'll be more prone to eating unhealthier foods since you need to pack all the nutrients that you need in just one meal.

The 16/8 Fasting Period

This protocol involve fasting for 16 hours with a feeding window of 8 hours. During the 8-hour period, dieters can eat a few meals, but the most ideal is eating the standard 3-meal a day. This is designed primarily for people who do weight training. It is also considered to be the most sophisticated form of intermittent fasting, and is the most popular form with athletes and bodybuilders.

Benefits: Aside from all the other benefits that you can get from fasting, 16/8 fast method offers excellent hormonal management. While other intermittent fasting protocols can provide that, only 16/8 offers daily increase of the growth hormone, thus maximizing the good effects of the growth hormone. This method does not alter your eating schedule the way the 20-hour and 24-hour methods do, so you don't experience the extreme hunger and low energy.

Drawbacks: This method is considered to be the most effective; hence, it is more of a hit than a miss. The only issue that might arise is if you aren't able to properly schedule your feeding and fasting times in to your regular schedule. It's recommended to start the fasting period when you go to sleep, and not begin the feeding period until 16 hours has passed.

Of the most popular protocols, the 16/8 method is probably the easiest and the most convenient. Since intermittent fasting is not a fad diet, but rather a lifestyle, it fits well into most people's daily routine. This is the method I would recommend to all, unless your schedule does not permit it.

Chapter 4 – Step-By-Step Guide to Intermittent Fasting

Intermittent fasting or periodically going without food for longer periods is an effective weight loss regimen that is different to any other diet menu plan, or weight loss fad.

Here is a step-by-step guide to help you begin intermittent fasting:

1. **Establish your goal/s.**

    It is important that you set your goals first before you even begin selecting the intermittent fasting protocol of your choice. Setting your goals gives you additional motivation to succeed. Here are some goals that you can consider:

    - *Lose body fat* – Isn't this one of the most important goals of most people who go on diets?

    - *Reduce eating time* – You can also substitute this with reducing the number of large meals.

    - *Increase levels of naturally-occurring growth hormone*, thereby increasing muscle, bone, and organ mass.

- *Increase immune functions* to increase your body's defense against infections and diseases.

2. Decide when to take your last meal.

Some people opt to decide whether they will begin their fasting period or not, on a daily basis. This may work for some, but it is better to put order to your regimen and set up a definite schedule. Plot on your virtual or physical calendar to work out the best system for you.

3. Do not just opt to "not eat" but also to change your diet.

Especially during the initial stages, you will experience the expected withdrawal and uncomfortable detoxification symptoms. You can alleviate these symptoms by altering your diet completely .You need to begin incorporating healthy foods, like fresh fruits and vegetables and lean meat; at the same time, cutting down on processed foods, soda, and red meat.

4. Avoid binging on your last meal.

Some people tend to binge-eat a little for their last meal. This is not a good practice because your body will only spend more time in food digestion rather than functioning and "adapting" to the fasting period. It defeats the purpose. Make sure that you eat the way you normally eat so you can maximize the benefits of intermittent fasting.

5. **Do not be in a hurry to get your hands (and mouth) on food.**

   Learn to patiently wait out on your fasting period. The main benefit of fasting is depriving your body of carbohydrates and calories. You can drink water during the fasting period; in fact, you can drink as much as you want. Light but healthy snacks may be allowed, but completely fasting is the optimum method.

Important Tips to Keep in Mind

When you are in your intermittent fasting regimen, keep the following in mind:

- Make sure you are properly hydrated because this is crucial in the detoxification process. It also keeps your body in an optimal state to heal itself.

- When you load up on a lot of carbohydrates during your last meal, you are highly likely to feel hungry early during your fasting period. Instead try and consume a meal higher in protein for your final meal.

- Expect initial discomfort and withdrawal symptoms, these are normal reactions of the body to the changes. Watch out for symptoms like headaches, vomiting and nausea, constipation, bloating, mental hunger, skin breakouts, and fatigue.

- Consult your doctor before you begin with intermittent fasting.

- If you have a history of eating disorders, you'll need to be extra careful. Just the same, consult a doctor and ask a family member or a friend to help you with the process. This ensures that you don't have a relapse of your previous condition.

- Pregnant women are not supposed to begin intermittent fasting.

Chapter 5 – Three Common Mistakes Made by Beginners

You have to realize that hunger is not the enemy. Make sure that you do not commit the following common mistakes when you begin with your intermittent fasting regimen:

- **Fear of getting hungry during the fasting period.**

    Face it, everybody gets hungry. It doesn't matter if you are under an intermittent fasting regimen or eating normally, you are bound to get hungry from time to time. Being hungry for a few hours should not be a huge concern. Some people, especially those who are beefing up their muscles, do not want to fast for fear that their muscle development will be jeopardized.

    The truth is your body could use the cleansing and detoxifying periods. What most people fail to realize is that the body can still function normally without eating even for 24 hours. When there is no intake of food, the body taps into your fat storage to utilize as energy for the body. Your body automatically burns fat when you don't "shove" food into it.

Just keep in mind that your digestive system could use a break.

- **Continuously eating unhealthy and junk foods.**

    In any case, whether you're eating the standard 6 meals a day or you are fasting, eating processed foods, junk foods, fast foods, and other unhealthy foods do not have a good effect on your body. You can't eat two bags of potato chips during your feeding period and assume that it's okay since you are going on a fasting period anyway. Intermittent fasting doesn't work that way, you still have to make sure that you eat healthy foods. Adding veggies, fruits, and healthy fats will work wonders. To lose weight, you still need to consume less calories than you burn every day. If you binge on unhealthy, calorie dense foods during your feeding period, you simply will not lose weight.

    Keep in mind that intermittent fasting does not give you the license to eat whatever you want just because you will be on a fasting period after. You cannot eat unhealthy foods, and expect to lose weight. It will never happen. It is important to practice some discipline because you will not be able to reach your goals without some hard work.

- **Counting the time to be able to finally binge.**

    Most beginners fail at intermittent fasting because they are prone to count the hours of their fasting periods. Keep in mind that fasting is not a fad diet, but a way of life. Your dedication and drive will propel you to successfully reach your goals. When you get worried about starving for a longer period of time, you have not fully understood what intermittent fasting is all about.

You don't have to be a "clock-watcher". You must learn to plan your fasting and feeding periods. Eat when the fast is over. You can adjust according to what fits your lifestyle. Do not force any scheduling scheme that would place you at a discomfort. Intermittent fasting has to fit perfectly right into your daily routine; it shouldn't control your schedule and your life. While it may seem difficult at first, eventually your body will adapt and you won't feel as hungry during your fasting periods.

Chapter 6 – Best Practices

Intermittent fasting is not just simply skipping meals and hoping you'll end up looking like a magazine pin-up model. The results may be appealing, but there are things that you need to consider to get the right results.

- **Your food choices are important.**

    Even if you are following a fasting regimen, you still have to consider the nutrients that you can get from the food you eat (when it's time to eat). You have to keep in mind the basic rules for good nutrition. When you fast for 20 hours and spend the next 4 hours of eating fast foods, like burgers and fries, you won't be able to get the results that you are hoping for.

- **Patience is a virtue.**

    One of the main thrusts of intermittent fasting is to skip breakfast, which is commonly considered to be the most important meal of the day. If you were used to eating breakfast, it will be a struggle for you, especially during the initial stages. You'll feel all the negative withdrawal symptoms, like morning moodiness, hunger pangs, and stomach rumblings. Despite the challenges, you have to draw strength from within so that you can pull through.

- **It won't hurt if you exercise.**

    Exercise is an integral part of the weight loss process; don't stop even if you are practicing intermittent fasting. Exercise complements this dieting pattern.

- **Establish a well-timed fasting schedule.**

    Whatever intermittent fasting protocol you follow, timing is the key to its success. You don't want to end up with a feeding window in the unholy hours of the morning, do you? To find what's best for you, try experimenting on the other fasting protocols.

- **Progress slowly.**

    Begin with an easy fasting/feeding schedule until you get the hang of it and you can eventually move to a more challenging protocol. Again, patience is the key. You cannot immediately jump into something you are not prepared for. When you have mastered the easy steps, you can move up to the more challenging protocols. Observe how your body reacts to the different intermittent fasting protocols and choose the one that you are most comfortable with.

- **Take it easy.**

    Be careful not to overdo it. You cannot get the results you want if you force it. Start slowly with a routine you can easily stick to.

- **You can eat meat.**

    You can still eat meat, don't think that you cannot. It is an excellent source of protein. But be careful to consume predominately lean meat.

- **Remember that intermittent fasting is a lifestyle, not a diet plan.**

    Compared to impossible-to-follow diet plans, intermittent fasting is more effective because it is a lifestyle. While you might encounter some difficulties in the beginning, when your body adapts to the routine of the feast/fast regimen, it will just be second nature to you. Soon, you won't even notice that you are in a special kind of regimen for losing weight.

- **Expect disapproving looks and reactions.**

    When you begin to skip breakfast, most people might not approve of it because of the meal's perceived importance. Disapproving reactions are normal; you don't need to get into arguments or intense discussions just to explain what you are doing. Don't waste your time explaining because some people won't be able to understand the method you have taken. You have to learn to live with that and soon they will understand what you have been working on.

- **Rehydrate.**

    Water is the best liquid for rehydration, but you can still drink tea or coffee (without milk and sugar) during your fasting period.

- **Some may be successful, some won't.**

    While everyone can try intermittent fasting, not everyone will be successful. There will be limitations, especially for those who have other medical conditions interfere with their fasting. Also, depending on people's schedules, home life, and drive, they will be prone to various levels of success.

    However, if you don't have any medical condition that will hinder your intermittent fasting regimen, you can always make the necessary adjustments (considering your other workable limitations), to ensure success.

- **Keep yourself busy.**

    Instead of watching every hour that passes during your fasting period, make yourself busy. Most beginners struggle with the waiting period. If you keep yourself busy, you are able to minimize the impact of the initial discomfort. For example, if you are on the 16/8 protocol, spend half of the 16 hours of fasting, sleeping, and then do other things around the house. You may begin a new hobby. Whatever you do to "kill time", it doesn't matter, as long as you stay as occupied as possible so you won't think about the fasting period. If your mind is constantly preoccupied, it won't send a signal to your body that you are hungry.

- **Don't expect miracles.**

While intermittent fasting can actually help you lose weight, along with its other benefits, that is just a single factor that will determine your overall health. Skipping breakfast or strictly following your chosen protocol can help you achieve your ideal weight. Other factors that will contribute to your overall well-being include eating healthy foods, and engaging in regular exercise. Fasting alone won't make you drop the excess weight, keep that in mind.

- **Do not over think.**

    Keep things simple. Intermittent fasting can help you lose weight; you just have to stay committed and driven. This is a simple lifestyle change, for the better. You'll encounter difficulties in the initial stages, do not panic and just be patient. Once your body gets used to the new routine, it will adapt to the regimen until it becomes second nature.

Intermittent fasting can give you positive benefits if you are trying to lose weight or build your muscles. There are several fasting protocols that you can choose from; the key is choosing the right fit for your daily routines.

Conclusion

Thank you again for downloading this book!

I hope this book was able to help you learn more about intermittent fasting.

The next step is to put this information to use, and begin implementing intermittent fasting in to your diet!

Remember to first consult a medical professional to ensure the routine you choose is suitable for your particular situation.

As previously mentioned, the 16/8 schedule is the most recommended routine, but it all depends on your particular schedule and lifestyle to what works best for you.

Finally, if you enjoyed this book, please take the time to share your thoughts and post a review on Amazon. It'd be greatly appreciated!

Thank you and good luck!

www.ingramcontent.com/pod-product-compliance
Lightning Source LLC
LaVergne TN
LVHW021747060526
838200LV00052B/3517